pocket**emergency medicine**

a quick
medical
reference
guide for use
on the wards

Gareth Rhys Chapman

First published 2010

1   2010
ISBN: 9781405193573

Catalogue records for this title are available from the British Library and
LOC.
Set in 7/8.5 Photina by Toppan Best-set Premedia Limited
Printed and bound in Singapore by Fabulous Printers Pte Ltd

Wiley-Blackwell makes no representation, express or implied, that the
drug dosages in this book are correct. Readers must therefore always
check that any product mentioned in this publication is used in accor-
dance with the prescribing information prepared by the manufacturers.
The author and the publishers do not accept responsibility or legal liabil-
ity for any errors in the text or for the misuse or misapplication of
material in this book.

Disclaimer: This is a guide only and management of patients
should not be based solely on the information contained within.
Please note that many lab values and treatment protocols vary by
trust/hospital/consultant and these should be confirmed.

Acknowledgements: I thank Dr Martina Toby, Dr Kirsty Dewar,
Dr Rachel Rolph, Dr James Duffy, Dr Sue Piper, Dr Janet Fallon,
Dr Emma Forsyth and Dr Tim Littlewood for their helpful comments and
advice in the compilation of this text.

Gareth Rhys Chapman

1 ABCDE

Follow the ABCDE approach when making the initial patient assessment.

Airway

Check airway is patent and maintained
- If the airway is difficult to maintain, consider manoeuvres (chin lift/jaw thrust) or the use of airway adjuncts, e.g. a Guedel airway
- If there is continued difficulty in maintaining an airway, fast bleep an anaesthetist, or put out a call for the cardiac arrest team

Breathing

Look, listen and feel for 10 seconds
- No pulse → call for cardiac arrest team
- No respiratory effort → call for cardiac arrest team
- To improve oxygen delivery to the tissues, consider giving supplementary oxygen
- Quickly auscultate for equal air entry and ensure the trachea is central. See Section 2 for further guidance on oxygen therapy

Circulation

- Obtain BP, pulse, temperature, O_2 sats, respiratory rate (RR), ECG
- Get a cannula in and take blood from it – see separate Sections on which bloods to send for each presentation
- If patient is shocked/hypotensive, commence IV fluids – see Section 2

Disability

Ensure the **BM** is checked (after ABC comes DEFG: Don't Ever Forget Glucose)
Undertake a rapid neurological assessment. AVPU is used in the critically ill patient:

A: alert; **V**: responds to vocal commands; **P**: responds to pain; **U**: unresponsive

If the patient is more stable, and you have longer to make an initial assessment, the Glasgow Coma Score (GCS) is a useful tool. A score of 8 or less indicates that intubation may be required:

Best motor response
6 – obeys commands; 5 – localises to pain; 4 – withdraws to pain; 3 – flexor response to pain; 2 – extensor response to pain; 1 – no response to pain

Best verbal response
5 – oriented; 4 – confused conversation; 3 – inappropriate speech; 2 – incomprehensible speech; 1 – no response

Eye opening
4 – spontaneous; 3 – open in response to speech; 2 – open in response to pain; 1 – no eye opening

Exposure – when A, B and C are managed

- Expose the patient, and search for any clues, e.g. signs of trauma, drug abuse, systemic illness, etc.
- Try to get some history: check the drug chart, check the patient's pockets for ID/Medicalert, question the relatives/nurses, read the initial clerking, ask for previous discharge summaries

If you are worried that the patient is deteriorating, ask for senior help early – people would rather be called to a peri-arrest than to an established one!

2 The breathless patient

- Ensure airway is patent and give supplementary oxygen
- Examine the patient, checking for signs of pneumothorax, infection, wheeze, absent breath sounds, heart failure
- Request a portable CXR (if the patient is unable to go to the department)
- Obtain IV access and take routine bloods, with cultures if you are considering initiating antibiotic therapy
- Undertake an ABG for vital information on oxygenation

Commonest symptoms/signs

Asthma	Wheeze
Pulmonary embolism	Pleuritic chest pain, sudden onset, possibly post-op/swollen calves, tachycardic
Tension pneumothorax	Reduced lung movement, agitated, distended neck veins, deviated trachea
Acute heart failure	Pink frothy sputum, raised JVP, chest creps
Pneumonia	Febrile, green/brown sputum, pleuritic chest pain
Infective exacerbation of COPD (IECOPD)	Pursed lips, accessory muscle use, productive cough, barrel chest

Acute respiratory failure: principles of oxygen therapy

Respiratory failure is when the P_aO_2 is <8 kPa. There are two types:
Type I: when the P_aCO_2 is low or within the normal range
Type II: when the P_aCO_2 is high (i.e. >6 kPa)
To tell the difference between types I and II you need to do an ABG

What will the patient look like?
In both types: short of breath, cyanosed (peripherally and possibly centrally – look around the mouth and at the tongue for pallor and a blue tinge); may be confused (less oxygen is getting to the brain). In type II the patient may also have a bounding, fast pulse, with a CO_2 retention flap at the wrist, and may complain of headache.

What is the immediate management?
Type I:
- High-flow oxygen via a face mask with a reservoir bag
- Aim for O_2 saturations of 94–98%
- Try to reverse the cause (which may be infection; acute events related to a chronic condition, e.g. COPD, asthma, trauma; or drugs)

Type II:
- **Be careful** giving oxygen therapy to these patients
- Use Venturi connectors to reduce the fraction of inspired oxygen to make sure you do not remove the drive to breathe
- Start with a blue connector (24% inspired oxygen), and increase if the patient does not improve – **hypoxia will kill before a reduced respiratory drive**, so do not be afraid to increase the concentration of inhaled oxygen. A good target for O_2 sats would be 88–92%
- Re-check the ABG after 1 hour (sooner if the GCS falls or the clinical picture alters significantly); if the P_aCO_2 levels are still rising despite oxygen

therapy, contact senior staff, as BiPAP/CPAP, respiratory stimulants and even intubation and ventilation may be required. If very frequent ABGs are required, consider asking senior staff to consider inserting an arterial line (but this may necessitate transfer to HDU/ITU)

Acute asthma

Acute, often reversible, exacerbation of a chronic airways disease, in which expiration is compromised more than inspiration.

What will the patient look like?
Wheezy, short of breath, anxious.

What is the immediate management?
Sit the patient up, give high-flow oxygen. To decide on further management, take pulse and RR, check O_2 sats, auscultate. Order a portable CXR (primarily to exclude pneumothorax). If the patient is able to carry out a peak flow test, do this (and ask what their normal peak flow value [PEF] is)

If RR is ≥25 breaths/min, pulse ≥110 beats/min, the PEF is <50% of best/predicted, or if the patient cannot complete sentences in one breath, the patient is having a **moderate to severe attack**:
- Give salbutamol 5 mg by oxygen-driven nebuliser
- Undertake an ABG: if the P_aCO_2 is normal or rising, this is a worrying sign, as is a falling pH; contact senior staff **immediately**
- If the patient is still no better after the nebuliser, start another 5-mg salbutamol nebuliser, and give prednisolone 40-50 mg p.o., or hydrocortisone 100 mg IV if the patient is unable to swallow
- If the patient remains unwell after a further 5 mins, contact senior staff again and explain that the patient is not improving
- Repeat salbutamol 5 mg with ipratropium 0.5 mg by O_2-driven nebuliser
- Consider continuous salbutamol nebuliser (5–10 mg/hour); senior staff may also suggest IV magnesium sulphate 1.2–2 g over 20 mins

If the PEF is <33% of best/predicted **or** there are **any** of SpO_2 <92%, silent chest/cyanosis, bradycardia/arrhythmia/low BP, or exhaustion, the patient is having a **life-threatening attack**:
- Contact senior staff and ITU **immediately**
- Ask the nurses to give salbutamol 5 mg and ipratropium 0.5 mg in the same high-flow oxygen-driven nebuliser, **and** prednisolone 40–50 mg p.o. or (if IV access is available) hydrocortisone 100 mg IV
- Undertake an ABG – if the P_aCO_2 is normal or rising, this is a worrying sign, as is a falling pH. If you are struggling with the ABG, do not persist whilst the patient's condition deteriorates
- If the patient remains unwell (i.e. sats remain poor, CO_2 is rising or GCS is falling), repeat the salbutamol and ipratropium nebuliser and contact senior staff again
- Consider continuous salbutamol nebuliser (5–10 mg/hour); senior staff may also suggest IV magnesium sulphate 1.2–2 g over 20 mins

If at any point a patient with a moderate to severe attack develops life-threatening symptoms, move immediately to the treatment algorithm for a life-threatening attack

Pulmonary embolism

Blood clot(s) from sites around the body (often the legs; deep vein thromboses [DVTs] dislodge, are pumped to the lungs, occluding circulation and causing a mismatch between ventilation and perfusion.

What will the patient look like?
Suddenly short of breath, often with pleuritic chest pain, possibly with haemoptysis and cyanosis. May present as sudden collapse in a post-operative patient.

What is the immediate management?
- ABCDE – see Section 1
- Give high-flow oxygen. Attach pulse oximeter
- If pain is a feature, give morphine 10 mg IV (vasodilator and anxiolytic) + metoclopramide 10 mg IV (antiemetic)
- Organise CXR, ABG, ECG
- Assess the probability of a pulmonary embolism (PE) – e.g., using Wells score (see below)
- If there is low to medium probability of a PE, undertake a D-dimer; if this is positive, or if there is a high probability of a PE **and** there is a normal CXR with no history of cardiorespiratory disease, proceed to a $\dot{V}/\dot{Q}$ scan; otherwise a CTPA is required
- Whilst awaiting the scan, commence low molecular weight heparin (LMWH) at treatment dose (e.g. enoxaparin 1.5 mg/kg)
- If hypotensive, start fluid replacement and liaise with HDU/ITU; thrombolysis may be required in the case of a large PE
- Once a diagnosis of PE is confirmed, warfarin will need to be started

Wells criteria for assessment of pre-test probability for PE

Feature	Score
Suspected DVT	3.0
Alternative diagnosis less likely than PE	3.0
Heart rate >100 bpm	1.5
Immobilisation/surgery in past 4 weeks	1.5
Previous DVT/PE	1.5
Haemoptysis	1.0
Malignancy (on treatment, treated within last 6 months, or palliative)	1.0

Score: <2: low probability; 2–6: medium probability; >6: high probability
Reproduced from *J Thromb Haemost*; Wells PS, Anderson DR et al.
83:416–20 (2000) with permission from Blackwell Publishing

Tension pneumothorax

Air within the pleural space, the amount increasing with each inspiration as air cannot escape during expiration; causes lung collapse and rapid progression to respiratory and cardiac arrest.

What will the patient look like?
Short of breath, very agitated, reduced chest movement on the affected side. The neck veins may be distended. The trachea may be deviated.

What is the immediate management?
- Ensure airway patency; give high-flow oxygen
- Quickly auscultate (reduced breath sounds on the affected side), feel for the trachea (deviated **away** from affected side), and percuss (hyper-resonant on affected side)
- Do **not** arrange any investigations at this stage
- Immediately insert a large-bore cannula (orange/brown/grey) into the *second intercostal space* just above the rib, in the *mid-clavicular line*. Remove the needle, but keep the cannula *in situ*. A hiss of air should be heard
- Contact senior staff to insert a chest drain; arrange a CXR

Acute heart failure
Acute failure of the pumping function of the heart (primarily left ventricular) causing significant pulmonary oedema.

What will the patient look like?
Short of breath – worse on lying, with pink, frothy sputum being produced. Physical signs include raised JVP, pulsus alternans, a third heart sound and pitting oedema. The patient may give a history of congestive heart failure, e.g. ankle swelling, decreased exercise tolerance, angina.

What is the acute treatment?
- ABCDE – see Section 1
- High-flow oxygen, with the patient as upright in bed as possible
- Obtain IV access, taking blood at the same time for U&E, FBC, and troponin, and attach cardiac monitors and pulse oximeter. Consider urinary catheterisation to monitor fluid balance. Obtain an ECG
- Give furosemide 40–80 mg IV slowly over 5–10 mins (vasodilator and diuretic), plus two puffs of GTN spray if SBP is >90 mmHg (vasodilator)
- If the patient is still no better, consider giving a further dose of furosemide, and contact senior staff – it may be necessary to start a nitrate infusion
- If you think the patient is experiencing an acute coronary syndrome, start ACS treatment (see Section 7)
- Organise a repeat troponin at 12 hours after the onset of symptoms

Pneumonia
A chest infection due to one of several causative organisms, which may be community or hospital acquired.

What will the patient look like?
Pale or flushed, sweating and short of breath, with a fever, cough that is productive of green/brown sputum, and often pleuritic chest pain.

What is the acute treatment?
- ABCDE – see Section 1
- Give high-flow oxygen, obtain IV access, and send blood for cultures, FBC, U&E, CRP, LFTs. Obtain a sputum sample and send for culture
- IV fluids to counter hypotension/dehydration, plus analgesia

- Stratify risk using the CURB-65 score:

Confusion (if AMTS score ≤8)	1 point
Urea concentration >7 mmol/L	1 point
RR ≥30 breaths/min	1 point
BP <90/60 mmHg	1 point
Age ≥**65** years	1 point

  Score: **0** or **1**: patient may be treated in the community – mild infection;
  2: inpatient therapy required – **moderate** infection; **3**+: inpatient therapy
  required – **severe** infection
- Determine if infection is hospital or community acquired:
  - community acquired = admitted from home or becomes unwell within
    first 48 hours of hospital admission
  - hospital acquired = becomes unwell >48 hours after admission
- Start antibiotic therapy – local guidelines vary according to the severity
  and type (hospital vs community) of pneumonia. Consult the microbiology
  department of your hospital without delay for prescribing information

Infective exacerbation of COPD
An acute deterioration of existing chronic airways disease, worsening the
patient's (already limited) respiratory function.

What will the patient look like?
Patient may be hunched over, using accessory muscles to aid with respira-
tion, cyanosed and appear gasping for breath, exhaling using pursed lips.

What is the acute treatment?
- ABCDE – see Section 1
- Controlled oxygen therapy using Venturi connectors (blue or white initially), aiming for saturations of 88–92% and to increase the P_aO_2 above
  8 kPa in most instances. Some patients, however, will have a normal base-
  line much lower than this, so ask the patient what their baseline is, or for
  a respiratory passport, which will provide a lot of useful information
- Start salbutamol 5 mg and ipratropium bromide 0.5 mg nebulisers
  (air-driven if known to be a CO_2 retainer), whilst requesting a CXR
  (confirms infection and excludes pneumothorax)
- Take blood for U&E, FBC, CRP and cultures
- Obtain a sputum sample for culture
- An ABG will allow you to see rapidly the severity of the exacerbation
- Begin 30 mg of prednisolone o.d. p.o.
- After taking cultures, commence antibiotics according to local guidelines
  (NICE recommends antibiotic therapy if there is a history of purulent
  sputum, consolidation on a CXR, or clinical evidence of pneumonia)
- If the patient is not improving after 5 mins of the previous nebulisers
  ending, start another salbutamol 5 mg and ipratropium bromide 0.5 mg
  nebuliser, and repeat the ABG
- If required, salbutamol nebulisers can be given back-to-back
- Contact senior staff, as IV aminophylline, as well as CPAP/BiPAP may be
  required at this stage

3 Hypotension/falling blood pressure
Commonest symptoms/signs

Key signs of shock	Tachycardia, hypotension, tachypnoea
Septic shock	Hypotensive, tachycardic, decreased GCS, usually in a febrile patient
Anaphylactic shock	Acute onset of facial swelling +/– stridor and signs of shock
Upper GI bleed	Haematemesis, melaena, hypotensive, tachycardic
Ruptured aortic aneurysm	Abdominal pain radiating to back; expansile, pulsatile abdominal mass, with signs of shock
Aortic dissection	Severe tearing chest pain, differing BPs in the arms, shocked, radio-radial delay
Cardiac tamponade	Raised JVP, muffled heart sounds, in shock

Septic shock

A significant and often overwhelming infection leading to severe systemic compromise of bodily functions. Vasodilatation is often extreme, causing severe hypotension and reduced organ perfusion.

What will the patient look like?

Usually hypotensive, tachycardic, decreased consciousness, tachypnoeic, febrile, with signs of a focus of infection (e.g. cough in pneumonia, dysuria in a UTI, wound dehiscence with wound site infection, etc.). The pulse may be bounding in character, and the patient may be peripherally very warm (due to vasodilatation).

What is the immediate management?

- ABCDE – see Section 1
- Give high-flow oxygen
- Obtain large-bore IV access in both antecubital fossae, and take blood for FBC, U&E, LFTs, CRP, cultures and clotting
- Give 1 L fluid stat (e.g. Hartmann's/normal saline/gelofusin)
- Perform a rapid assessment of the patient, searching for an obvious sign of sepsis, and referring to the notes where available. If a source is found, culture it (e.g. wound swabs/skin swabs) and remove if possible (e.g. take out infected lines)
- If the chest is a possible source of sepsis, request a CXR
- Do an ABG to obtain information on the pH, oxygenation, and lactate levels
- Undertake a urine dip; send sample for culture
- Consider catheterisation to aid with fluid balance. Ask nursing staff to keep a strict fluid balance chart
- Start empirical antibiotics against the presumed source of sepsis; these will vary according to your local policy, usually available on the local intranet. These should be started **within the first hour** of recognising severe sepsis
- If no source of sepsis is identified, broad-spectrum antibiotics can be initiated

- Call senior staff to inform them of the steps you have undertaken; the patient may deteriorate rapidly and may require HDU/ITU input
- If no clear source of sepsis is found, consider an echocardiogram (?vegetations), or imaging (e.g. ultrasound scan in ?biliary sepsis)

Anaphylactic shock

An allergic response leading to release of large amounts of immunological factors and causing oedema and vasodilatation. Common precipitants include bee stings, peanuts and drugs.

What will the patient look like?

The patient may appear oedematous and flushed, there may be a rash, and the patient may be breathless with a wheeze or stridor. Patient is likely be tachycardic and hypotensive.

What is the immediate management?
- ABCDE – see Section 1; ongoing oedematous reaction can mean that the airway is compromised early. If there are any signs of swelling/wheeze/stridor, contact an anaesthetist immediately to intubate
- Give high-flow oxygen
- Quickly try to identify and remove the source (look at the drug chart, examine around the bed, stop any infusions)
- Give adrenaline 0.5 mg (i.e. 0.5 mL of a 1:1000 solution) IM: **this concentration, dose and route is different to that used in a cardiac arrest – ensure you double check the ampoule before administration**
- Ask the nurse to connect the patient to a cardiac monitor, preferably with a defibrillator available, and re-check observations every 5 mins
- Obtain large-bore IV access; give fluids (1 L normal saline stat)
- Give hydrocortisone 200 mg IV and chlorphenamine (Piriton) 10 mg IV
- Call senior staff. If there is no improvement, continue with IM adrenaline boluses every 5 mins. Salbutamol 5 mg nebulisers driven with high-flow oxygen may replace the wheeze

Large upper GI bleed

Bleeding from the upper part of the gastrointestinal tract.

What will the patient look like?

The patient will be peripherally shut-down, tachycardic, hypotensive, oliguric and have a postural BP drop. There will be a history of haematemesis and/or melaena; they may have known varices. There may be epigastric pain, and the patient may appear clinically anaemic.

What is the immediate management?
- ABCDE – see Section 1; ensure there are no blood clots occluding the airway
- Give high-flow oxygen
- Obtain large-bore venous access in both antecubital fossae; take urgent bloods for FBC, U&E, LFTs, clotting and an urgent cross-match for 6 units
- Give 1 L gelofusin/Hartmann's/normal saline stat initially
- Catheterise the patient; start a strict fluid balance chart

- Contact senior staff, who may ask for the Rockall score, which stratifies risk. A copy of the pre-endoscopy (modified) Rockall score is given below. Ask if you should prescribe a PPI (e.g. pantoprazole)
- If the patient remains compromised, give blood (O negative if cross-matched blood is not yet available)
- Undertake regular observations; ensure Hb is checked regularly (e.g. 2 hours post-transfusion); further units' transfusion may be required
- A central line may become necessary to guide volume replacement
- An urgent endoscopy is required. If bleed is significant, ensure the surgeons are informed

Pre-endoscopy modified Rockall score (max. 7 points)

	0 points	1 point	2 points	3 points
Age (years)	<60	60–79	80+	
Shock:				
SBP	>100 mmHg	>100 mmHg	<100 mmHg	
Heart rate	<100 bpm	>100 bpm		
Co-morbidity	No major co-morbidities	IHD Cardiac failure	Liver failure Renal failure	Metastatic carcinoma

Ruptured abdominal aortic aneursym

A dilated aorta in the patient's abdomen ruptures, causing catastrophic blood loss and decreased perfusion to vital organs.

What will the patient look like?

The patient will be very unwell. Abdominal pain will radiate to the back, the patient will be tachycardic and hypotensive, as well as peripherally shut down. There may well be an expansile, pulsatile mass in the epigastrium.

What is the immediate management?
- ABCDE – see Section 1
- Give oxygen
- Ask a nurse to fast-bleep a surgeon (preferably vascular) and your registrar immediately
- Obtain wide-bore IV access; take blood for FBC, U&E, amylase; cross-match for 8–10 units
- Do not blindly give fluids, but **monitor BP closely** – the aim is to maintain organ perfusion, not to make the patient normotensive: even a normal systolic blood pressure could lead to a catastrophic increase in intra-abdominal bleeding. Replace volume only when absolutely necessary (i.e. to maintain consciousness) with gelofusin or O negative blood until cross-matched blood becomes available

Acute aortic dissection

This occurs when the wall of the aorta tears, causing a false lumen to present, and meaning that blood flow is diverted away from the vessels supplied by the aorta into the new lumen. Type A dissections involve the ascending aorta; type B dissections are distal to the left subclavian artery.

What will the patient look like?
The patient will complain of a severe tearing pain in the centre of the chest or between the scapulae; will often be tachycardic, hypotensive and dizzy, and will most likely have a radio-radial delay, and differing blood pressure in each arm.

What is the immediate management?
- ABCDE – see Section 1
- Give high-flow oxygen
- Obtain wide-bore IV access; take blood for FBC, U&E, amylase; cross-match for 8–10 units
- Request an ECG to exclude other causes of chest pain
- Give subcutaneous morphine 5–10 mg with 10 mg IV metoclopramide
- Contact senior staff who may request imaging, e.g. CT/MRI, or rapid surgery

Cardiac tamponade
Fluid accumulates in the sac surrounding the heart, leading to impairment in function and embarrassment of the circulation. It may be due to trauma, dissection, malignancy, infection, or a recent MI.

What will the patient look like?
The patient will be in shock with tachycardia and hypotension. JVP will be raised with an abnormal waveform (rises on inspiration) and possibly muffled heart sounds. The triad of increased CVP, hypotension and quiet heart sounds is known as Beck's triad.

What is the immediate management?
- ABCDE – see Section 1
- Give high-flow oxygen
- Obtain IV access – give fluids (colloid) if patient is significantly hypotensive
- Discuss urgently with senior staff – an emergency pericardiocentesis may be required
- An ECG may be helpful, and will demonstrate small complexes; it can also exclude ongoing cardiac ischaemia/infarction. CXR will show a large circular heart. An echo is diagnostic

4 Disordered consciousness
Commonest symptoms/signs

Meningitis	Photophobia, neck stiffness, temperature, possible rash
Subarachnoid haemorrhage	Thunderclap occipital headache, sometimes followed by drowsiness
Stroke	New onset of sensory or motor deficits that do not resolve rapidly
Status epilepticus	Fitting, with tongue biting, urinary incontinence
Metabolic events/poisons	See Sections 5&6

Meningitis
Infection and swelling of the meninges (coverings of the brain and CNS).

What will the patient look like?
Confused or decreased consciousness, febrile, avoids light, stiff neck, ? rash.

What is the immediate management?
- ABCDE – see Section 1
- IV access and rapid fluids (saline or gelofusin); take bloods for FBC, U&E, cultures; give high-flow oxygen
- Antibiotics (e.g. ceftriaxone 2 g IV b.d.) are urgently required and vary according to local guidelines.
- Contact senior staff urgently in case they wish to undertake a lumbar puncture prior to giving antibiotics (usually preceded by a CT in the case of a decreased GCS). **If you cannot get hold of senior staff rapidly, do not delay giving antibiotics**
- Do not forget that it is your duty to ensure Public Health are informed of the case – household contacts will require prophylaxis

Subarachnoid haemorrhage
Sudden bleed into the subarachnoid space, e.g. from an aneurysmal source.

What will the patient look like?
The patient will probably complain of a sudden 'thunderclap' occipital headache, associated with collapse ± vomiting and coma. There may also be focal neurology and signs of meningism.

What is the immediate management?
- ABCDE – see Section 1
- Urgent CT scan; an urgent neurosurgical opinion may be necessary
- In the interim, start the patient on neurological observations
- If the CT is negative but the patient remains ill and the history remains suggestive of a bleed, contact senior staff to conduct an LP (remember to look for xanthochromia)

Stroke
There are two main types: **ischaemic** (usually due to occlusion by a thrombus of cardiac or carotid artery origin) or **haemorrhagic** (usually due to aneurysmal rupture or hypertension).

What will the patient look like?

This depends on where the stroke affects: **cerebral hemisphere:** classical hemiplegia with speech problems if Broca's/Wernicke's areas are affected; **lacunar:** deficits vary from pure motor/sensory to mixed signs; **brainstem:** symptoms vary and may include involvement of all four limbs, and cranial nerves. e.g. gaze palsies

What is the immediate management?

- ABCDE – see Section 1
- Nil by mouth (NBM) and IV access. Give fluids for hydration
- **Do not** acutely lower blood pressure, unless systolic BP is >220 mmHg, and even then, only do so under expert guidance. Raised BP is the body's protection mechanism to limit brain injury
- A CT scan is vital – this allows haemorrhagic and ischaemic strokes to be differentiated. Blood is white on a CT for up to 7 days after the bleed
- If an ischaemic stroke is diagnosed, give aspirin 300 mg o.d.. If onset of symptoms was in the last 3 hours, contact senior staff as they may wish to thrombolyse with t-PA
- If a haemorrhagic stroke is diagnosed, **stop** any anticoagulation; involve senior staff – a neurosurgical opinion will likely be sought; a raised INR may need to be reversed using e.g. vitamin K – ask senior staff
- Admit patient to a stroke unit – outcomes are better; arrange an echo and carotid dopplers to seek a source of emboli

Status epilepticus

Either one prolonged seizure lasting >30 mins, or several seizures in quick succession without full recovery between seizures.

What will the patient look like?

Usually unconscious, fitting, may have wet themselves or have blood around the mouth from a bitten tongue.

What is the immediate management?

- ABCDE – see Section 1. Airway manoeuvres may be difficult but attempt to insert a Guedel or nasopharyngeal airway. Suction may be helpful
- Place the patient in the recovery position and remove anything obvious that may injure the patient (e.g. table, drip stand); if the patient is in bed raise the cot sides, which can be cushioned with pillows
- Ask a nurse to carry out serial observations, and check BMs – give glucose stat if low (see Section 5)
- Attempt cannulation, take blood, including for anti-convulsant levels if patient is a known epileptic
- Give lorazepam 2–4 mg IV or diazepam 5–10 mg per rectum
- If the patient is a known alcoholic, give parenteral thiamine
- When safe to do so, examine the patient for any signs of illness (especially infection) that may have precipitated the fit; call for senior help
- If the patient is still fitting after 10 mins, repeat 2–4 mg IV **or** diazepam 5–10 mg per rectum, and call an anaesthetist – the next step is to start phenytoin, phenobarbitol or even thiopental infusion

5 Metabolic emergencies
Commonest symptoms/signs

DKA	Deep, sighing breathing, with 'sweet-smelling' breath
HONK	Very dehydrated, usually elderly patient, not necessarily previously known to be diabetic
Hypoglycaemia	Low GCS, confused, possibly fitting
Hyperkalaemia	May be well; high K^+ on bloods

Diabetic ketoacidosis (DKA)

Usually presents as high sugar levels in a type 1 diabetic, with acidosis on ABG, and ketone production.

What will the patient look like?

Usually drowsy or unconscious with 'sweet-smelling' breath (ketones), hyperventilation, and sometimes abdominal pains with vomiting. The patient is invariably very dehydrated.

What is the immediate management?
- ABCDE – see Section 1
- Check BM
- Ask a nurse to dipstick the urine
- Obtain IV access, take bloods (including a lab glucose as a double-check, and U&Es to monitor K^+); undertake cultures (as infection often precipitates DKA); check amylase if patient has abdominal pain
- Undertake an ABG to assess pH (get senior help if pH < 7, whilst carrying out the management plan below; senior staff may give sodium bicarbonate, but you should never give this without senior instruction)
- Start IV normal saline: give the first bag stat, the second over 1 hour, then reassess fluid status (catheterisation will help with this); subsequent bags should be given 2- to 4-hourly until hypovolaemia is corrected, with a switch to 5% dextrose when BMs <12
- Start an insulin sliding scale: local guidelines vary but here is an example:

BM – check hourly	Insulin (as IV infusion of, e.g., Actrapid)
Under 4	Call doctor
4–7	1 unit/hour
7.1–11	2 units/hour
11.1–20	4 units/hour
Over 20	Give 7 units/hour, then call doctor

- Aim for a reduction in BMs of about 3 mmol/hour
- Give prophylactic LMWH, e.g. enoxaparin 40 mg subcut. (check local guidelines)
- Consider antibiotics as sepsis may have precipitated, or be complicating, the situation
- Continue with venous gases 4-hourly (for pH/lactate levels). Check the K^+ level on the gas – replace even when the K^+ concentration is in the normal range, as insulin causes K^+ to migrate intracellularly. Monitor BMs hourly until the patient is stable

Hyperosmolar non-ketotic state (HONK)

Very high sugars in a type 2 diabetic, with a very high plasma osmolality $[2(Na^+ + K^+) + urea + glucose$; upper limit of normal 299 mmol/L], but no ketones.

What will the patient look like?
Usually elderly, the onset is less acute than with DKA, and the patient will be very dehydrated.

What is the immediate management?
- ABCDE – see Section 1
- Check BM
- Ask a nurse to dipstick the urine; patients with HONK may still have up to ketones ++ on a dip. A blood ketone meter will help to exclude the presence of ketones in the blood and hence will exclude a DKA
- Obtain IV access, take bloods (including a lab glucose as a double-check, U&E, FBC, CRP), and undertake cultures (as infection may precipitate HONK)
- Give normal saline **alone** over 30 min
- Give treatment dose LMWH (if not in renal failure)
- Repeat the bag of normal saline – again over 30 min – and check BMs
- Aim for a reduction in BMs of about 3 mmol/hour
- If no response on just fluids, give 1 unit of insulin over 1 hour. Continue fluids at a rate of 1 L/hour
- If still an inadequate response, start on an insulin sliding scale; local guidelines vary but here is an example:

BM – check hourly	Insulin (as IV infusion of, e.g., Actrapid)
Under 4	Call doctor
4–7	1 unit/hour
7.1–11	2 units/hour
11.1–20	3 units/hour
Over 20	Give 4 units/hour, then call doctor

Often type 2 diabetics are exquisitely sensitive to insulin – BMs may fall rapidly, so keep a close eye!
- Consider antibiotics as sepsis may have precipitated, or be complicating, the situation

Hypoglycaemia

Low blood sugar; BMs <3.5

What will the patient look like?
The patient will often have reduced consciousness, may be tachycardic and confused, possibly aggressive.

What is the immediate management?
- Ensure the airway is patent, and protect if necessary
- Check BM and assess GCS
- If the patient *does not* have a low consciousness level, i.e. swallow is intact, give HypoStop/Lucozade orally, along with slow-release sugars (e.g.

biscuits). Continue to monitor BMs until persistently within the normal range (>4)

- If the patient *does* have a low consciousness level, i.e. swallow is not intact, carry out management as below:
- ABCDE – see Section 1
- Obtain venous access, send off bloods – do not forget to request a lab glucose
- Give 50 mL 50% dextrose, with a good flush (dextrose is irritant to the veins); if 20% dextrose is readily available, give 200 mL of this **instead** of the 50% solution, as there is less risk of tissue damage
- If you are unable to obtain venous access, an alternative is glucagon 1 mg IM (give this injection once only)
- The patient should recover in a matter of minutes rather than hours; consider an IV infusion of dextrose (5% or even 10%) if sugars continue to run low, after discussion with a specialist
- Continue to monitor BMs until persistently within the normal range (>4)
- Review regular medication: oral diabetic drugs may need to be withheld or dosage decreased

Hyperkalaemia

High levels of K^+ in the serum: >6.5 mmol/L or >5.5 mmol/L with ECG changes.

What will the patient look like?
The patient may appear well. Blood tests will show a high K^+, and there may be ECG changes of: tented, tall T-waves; broad QRS complexes; flattened P waves.

What is the immediate management?
- Cardiac monitoring is essential
- Obtain venous access; take bloods, sending off an urgent U&E. Take some blood to a blood gas analyser for an immediate K^+ reading, as falsely high K^+ readings from lab samples are common due to haemolysis and potassium leaking from cells
- If K^+ >6.5, or ECG changes exist, give 10 mL of 10% calcium gluconate over 2 mins, to protect the cardiac myocardium
- Give 10 units of Actrapid in 50 mL 50% dextrose as an IV infusion over 10 mins
- Assess fluid status. If patient is fluid depleted, rehydration is essential to aid with urinary K^+ excretion
- Call for senior advice: you may be asked to give calcium resonium (a longer acting potassium binder) or salbutamol nebulisers
- Ensure that K^+ is re-checked and followed up on regularly over the next few hours; levels may increase again after initial management
- Halt any drugs (e.g. potassium-sparing diuretics) that may lead to hyperkalaemia

6 Poisoning
Commonest symptoms/signs

Paracetamol overdose	Often nil within first 24 hours
Opiate overdose	Low GCS, 'pinpoint' pupils, low RR
Aspirin overdose	Vomiting, dehydration, dizziness, tinnitus
Tricyclic antidepressant overdose	Dilated pupils with blurred vision, tachycardia, dry mouth

National Poisons Bureau: 0844 892 0111

A note on gastric lavage and activated charcoal
- Gastric lavage is rarely used, but can be considered within the first hour following overdose. It involves passing a tube into the stomach and literally washing out the contents to prevent further absorption of toxins. It should be undertaken only with senior guidance
- Activated charcoal is more widely used. Toxins are adsorbed onto the charcoal surface, resulting in reduced uptake into the body. The adult dose is 50 g diluted in water for oral consumption. Local guidelines will state the time until which charcoal can be prescribed following an overdose

Paracetamol overdose
Ingestion of paracetamol, or paracetamol-containing products, over and above the normal dose (1 g q.d.s for adults). In adults, 12 g may be fatal.

What will the patient look like?
Often the patient will appear well. After about 24 hours, symptoms of right upper quadrant pain, jaundice and nausea/vomiting may occur.

What is the immediate management?
- ABCDE – see Section 1
- Obtain venous access; take blood, in particular for U&E, LFTs and clotting (including an INR). If the overdose was taken within the last 4 hours, take blood again at the 4-hour mark for paracetamol and salicylate levels. If the overdose was taken *more* than 4 hours ago, send off bloods for these levels immediately
- Obtain a full history, especially amount taken and when; if the tablets were taken with any alcohol/other drugs; previous overdoses; previous medical and drug history; social history
- If the patient tries to self-discharge, contact senior staff – the patient may require forcible admission under the Mental Capacity Act
- When the blood level is back, check the level on the treatment graph opposite.
- Give Parvolex (i.e. acetylcysteine) if the result is **on or above** the treatment line, to the following schedule:
  - 150 mg/kg in 200 mL 5% dextrose over 15 mins as an IV infusion; then:
  - 50 mg/kg in 500 mL 5% dextrose over 4 hours as an IV infusion; then:
  - 100 mg/kg in 1 L 5% dextrose over 16 hours as an IV infusion
- A rash is a common side effect of Parvolex treatment – do not stop the infusion simply because a rash presents; however, be alert to signs of anaphylaxis (see Section 3)

Paracetamol treatment curve

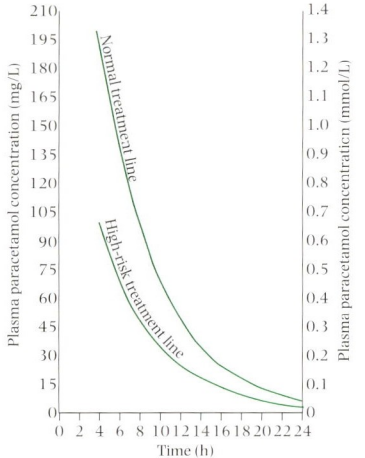

NB: The high-risk treatment line is for patients who are malnourished or receiving enzyme-inducing drugs

- If the patient weighs over 110 kg (17 stones), use 110 kg as body weight in the above calculations to avoid acetylcysteine toxicity
- Submit a blood request for an INR after the course of Parvolex: if the INR is >1.4, discuss with senior staff (may require further Parvolex)

Opiate overdose

Ingestion of excessive amounts of heroin, methadone or morphine-based drugs. May be iatrogenic.

What will the patient look like?
Often decreased consciousness, 'pinpoint' pupils, and decreased RR and effort. Patient may show signs of intravenous drug use (abscesses, injection marks, unkempt), or may be a known terminally ill or post-operative patient (on opiate-based analgesics).

What is the immediate management?
- ABCDE – see Section 1
- Give high-flow oxygen, monitor O_2 sats
- Obtain venous access; take baseline bloods, including FBC, U&E, LFTs
- Give naloxone 400 micrograms IV (if IV unavailable, give IM)
- Naloxone effects last for only a couple of minutes; if GCS starts to fall again after initial administration of naloxone, repeat the dose every 2–3 mins, until the patient is more alert and RR rises. A continuous infusion of naloxone may become necessary

- Consider ABG if RR remains low – is your diagnosis correct?
- Obtain a sample of urine for drug screen to confirm presence of opiates

Aspirin (salicylate) overdose

Ingestion of aspirin or aspirin-containing products above the normal dose.

What will the patient look like?

Dehydrated, vomiting, dizzy (due to vertigo), sweaty; may complain of ringing in the ears (tinnitus).

What is the immediate management?

- ABCDE – see Section 1
- Obtain venous access; take blood, especially for salicylate and paracetamol levels, LFTs, U&E and INR
- Undertake an ABG – the patient is at risk of developing a respiratory alkalosis
- Check BM regularly
- Consider catheterisation; ask nurses to regularly dip the urine for pH
- Contact senior staff, who may want to give sodium bicarbonate or undertake alkalinisation of the urine

Tricyclic antidepressant (TCA) overdose

Ingestion of TCAs over and above the normal dose. TCA examples: amitriptyline, clomipramine and trimipramine. TCAs have a narrow therapeutic window, so relatively small overdoses can lead to significant toxicity.

What will the patient look like?

The patient may well have dilated pupils with blurred vision, a dry mouth, possibly drowsiness, tachycardia, hyper-reflexia and urinary retention.

What is the immediate management?

- ABCDE – see Section 1
- Obtain venous access; send off blood for FBC, U&E, LFTs, salicylate and paracetamol levels, as well as specific levels for the drug ingested (discuss with the lab)
- Attach the patient to a cardiac monitor, and obtain a 12-lead ECG – arrhythmias are very common, including broad QRS, prolonged PR, as well as heart block
- Give IV fluids if hypotension is a feature
- Undertake an ABG
- Call senior staff with the above results to hand

7 Low urine output
Commonest symptoms/signs

Pre-renal renal failure | Underfilled: low JVP, dry mucous membranes, decreased BP, tachycardic

Post-renal renal failure | Fluid status may appear normal; suprapubic discomfort

There are many intrinsic causes of renal failure. If the cause does not appear to be pre- or post-renal, do not forget to consider other causes.

Pre-renal renal failure

By far the commonest cause of decreased urine output – usually underfilling, due to dehydration or excessive diuretic use.

What will the patient look like?

Urine output <0.5 mL/kg/hour. The patient will generally look dry, with dry mucous membranes, non-visible JVP, prolonged CRT (capillary refill time) and cool peripheries. They may well be tachycardic and hypotensive.

What is the immediate management?

- Firstly, assess fluid status. Look at the mucous membranes, check the JVP, check the BP and heart rate. Quickly read through the clerking/operation notes. Look at the fluid balance chart (if present). Listen to the lung bases and feel for pitting ankle oedema
- Cannulate the patient and take bloods, especially for U&Es. A venous blood gas may also be useful to assess for acidosis in the presence of renal failure
- Catheterisation allows you to keep a close eye on fluid output. If the patient is already catheterised, ask the nurses to flush the catheter to ensure the lumen is patent. If the patient is not catheterised, ask the nurses to do so
- If little urine comes out after catheterisation, or if the patient is already catheterised and the output is below 0.5 mL/kg/hour, ask the nurses to notate the obs, and then give 500 mL normal saline/Hartmann's stat. (If the patient is known to have cardiac failure (CCF), consider decreasing this to 250 mL)
- Repeat the obs. 5–10 mins after administration of the fluid; if matters have improved, you know that the patient was underfilled and requires replacement – a good starting point is 1 L over 2–4 hours
- If the obs. did not improve, it may be that the patient is in dire need of fluids (and so the little you have given has had barely any impact) or is already well-filled. Does the patient look dry? If so, give another bolus of 500 mL normal saline/Hartmann's (or 250 mL if known CCF), which will hopefully have an effect on the obs.
- If there is still no progress, contact senior staff, making sure you have the fluid balance chart, obs., and latest U&Es to hand

Post-renal renal failure

A blockage in the urinary tract after the kidney – may be due to tumour, blocked catheter, stone, or enlarged prostate.

What will the patient look like?
The patient will have a low urine output and may well be in a significant amount of discomfort (localised suprapubically).

What is the immediate management?
- Examine the patient. If there is suprapubic tenderness and a palpable bladder, the cause is most likely obstruction
- If a catheter is *in situ*, ask the nurses to flush it; if there is any impedance to flow, the catheter may need to be changed
- A bladder scanner is very useful at rapidly assessing the volume of urine in the bladder – ask the nurses to perform a scan if a scanner is available. If there is a large volume of urine in the bladder, there is likely an occlusion of the outflow tract
- If no catheter is in place, attempt to catheterise the patient
- If any urine is available, dip it, and send for microscopy, culture and sensitivities
- Take bloods, especially for U&Es. A venous blood gas may also be useful to assess for acidosis in the presence of renal failure. Consider sending blood cultures, as urine stagnating in the bladder is a potential source of sepsis
- Perform a PR in men to establish whether the prostate is enlarged (hence occluding the urinary tract)
- If you are unable to catheterise the patient, or if after catheterisation urine output remains poor, contact senior staff, who may ask for renal tract imaging ± suprapubic catheterisation. If you have never undertaken a suprapubic catheterisation, demand senior guidance – one paper quoted a 30-day mortality rate of 1.8% for this seemingly routine procedure![1]

[1] *Ann R Coll Surg Engl*; Anluwalia RS, Johal N *et al.* **88**:210–13 (2006)

8 Acute chest pain
Commonest symptoms/signs

ACS/MI	Central crushing chest pain, radiating to jaw/arm, nausea, clamminess
Pulmonary embolism	Pleuritic chest pain, sudden onset, possibly post-op; swollen calves, tachycardic
Aortic dissection	Severe tearing chest pain, differing BPs, shocked, radio-radial delay

Acute coronary syndrome (ACS)

Occlusion of the coronary arteries, leading to myocardial ischaemia and eventually myocardial death.

What will the patient look like?

The patient will complain of chest pain that is often central and 'crushing' – it may well radiate up into the jaw and down the arm(s). The patient will be sweaty, short of breath, and feel nauseous. If the patient has a degree of neuropathy (e.g. diabetics), the chest pain may be less obvious. Epigastric pain can sometimes occur during an MI.

What is the immediate management?
- ABCDE – see Section 1
- Give the **MONAC** drugs:
  - **M**orphine: 5–10 mg IV + **M**etoclopramide 10 mg IV
  - **O**xygen: high-flow via a non-re-breather bag
  - **N**itrates: i.e. GTN spray (two puffs or one tablet)
  - **A**spirin: 300 mg p.o.
  - **C**lopidogrel: 300 mg p.o. loading dose, with 75 mg p.o. daily thereafter
- Ask the nurses to obtain a 12-lead ECG and attach the patient to a cardiac monitor. Take serial ECGs (every 5–10 mins) to monitor any T wave changes. If possible, obtain old ECGs. Examine the patient, especially looking for a new murmur/signs of heart failure. Request a CXR to look for evidence of pulmonary oedema
- If there is ST elevation (>2 mm in 2+ contiguous chest lead, >1 mm in 2+ limb leads) or *new onset* LBBB, contact senior staff immediately, as the patient may require PCI (percutaneous coronary intervention) or thrombolysis. Remember, 1 mm is the equivalent of one small square on the ECG tracing
- If there is not ST elevation, this is likely an NSTEMI; ensure that the patient is on a full treatment dose of anticoagulation (e.g. enoxaparin 1 mg/kg b.d. subcut), and that the patient is on a beta-blocker (unless contraindicated, e.g. bradycardia/asthma) and aspirin (75 mg). Commence a statin (e.g. simvastatin 40 mg o.d.) unless already prescribed
- Contact senior staff; a GTN infusion ± angiography may be required, and the patient may need to be nursed in a coronary care unit
- Remember to order bloods for 12 hours after the onset of pain to measure the troponin level

Pulmonary embolism: See Section 2
Aortic dissection: See Section 3

9 The acute abdomen

There are many causes of an acute abdomen; this section does not aim to be exhaustive, but provides guidance in managing some of the *commonest* causes.

Commonest symptoms/signs

Appendicitis	Periumbilical/right iliac fossa pain, low-grade fever
Acute pancreatitis	Epigastric pain, radiating to back
Perforated peptic ulcer	Epigastric pain, guarding, rigidity
Intestinal obstruction	Abdominal pain, constipation, distension, vomiting
Renal colic	Loin-to-groin pain
Ectopic pregnancy	Female of child-bearing age with unilateral iliac fossa pain
Acute cholecystitis	Right upper quadrant (RUQ)/epigastric pain, Murphy's +ve, nausea, febrile
Constipation	Generalised abdominal pains, bowels not opened for several days, or diarrhoea with faecal loading

Appendicitis

Inflammation of the appendix, causing acute pain.

What will the patient look like?

The patient will usually complain of pain that starts periumbilically, but which migrates to the right iliac fossa. Low-grade fever and tachycardia are often present. There is rebound tenderness and localised guarding; movement exacerbates the pain.

What is the immediate management?

- An appendicectomy is often necessary, so contact a surgeon early
- Meanwhile, take blood for FBC, U&E, LFTs, amylase, clotting, ESR, CRP, cultures
- Obtain a urine sample: dip for UTI, and exclude pregnancy
- Do a group and save, as the patient will likely go for surgery
- Make the patient NBM, and give fluids. When did the patient last eat?
- Request an erect CXR and an AXR to exclude other causes of acute abdomen; ask the surgeons if they would like an USS (note this is often not diagnostic). Request an ECG (for the anaesthetists' pre-op assessment)
- Start antibiotics (local policies vary; an example would be both metronidazole 500 mg tds and cefuroxime 1.5 g tds – both IV), unless the diagnosis is unclear, in which case a period of 'watchful waiting' is often employed
- Reassess often – place on regular obs with clear instructions to call you if the patient begins to deteriorate

Acute pancreatitis

Inflammation of the pancreas, most often due to gallstones or alcohol.

What will the patient look like?

The patient will complain of pain centred in the epigastrium that bores through to the back. The patient is often dry, and may vomit, leading to shock, with tachycardia, fever and peritonitic abdomen. Later, there may be bruising of the flanks or periumbilically. The patient can become very ill, and may require ITU intervention – consider this early.

What is the immediate management?

- ABCDE – see Section 1
- IV access and fluids (normal saline/Hartmann's). Make the patient NBM. Send bloods for FBC, U&E, Ca^{2+}, LFTs, clotting, amylase (usually raised in the acute phase of pancreatitis), lipase (if available), cultures (if febrile), and CRP. Ask for a BM to be done (if high, consider sliding scale)
- Undertake an ABG – focus on pH and pO_2
- Erect CXR/AXR to exclude other causes of acute abdomen
- Ask for a strict fluid balance chart – if there are any concerns, consider catheterisation; these patients often require large amounts of fluid due to third-spacing
- Write up prn morphine, with regular paracetamol and anti-emetic (e.g. cyclizine 50 mg tds p.o./IV/IM)
- Calculate a severity score for prognostication and deciding the most appropriate setting for continued care (i.e. is transfer to ITU appropriate?):

Modified Glasgow Criteria ('PANCREAS')

PaO₂	<8 kPa
Age	>55 years
Neutrophils	WBC > 15 × 10⁹/L
Calcium	<2 mmol/L
Renal function	Urea >16 mmol/L
Enzymes	LDH >600 iu/L; AST >200 iu/L
Albumin	<32 g/L
Sugar (i.e. blood glucose)	>10 mmol/L

Score 1 point for each of the above
A score ≥3 indicates ITU care may well be appropriate

- Contact senior staff who may request USS/CT/MRCP/ERCP

Perforated peptic ulcer

When an ulcer in the stomach or duodenum erodes through the gut wall.

What will the patient look like?

Usually lying still, in large amount of (initially epigastric) pain with tachycardia and tachypnoea; often nauseous. The patient may demonstrate shallow breathing, and upon palpation the abdomen will be very tender, with guarding and rigidity.

What is the immediate management?

- ABCDE – see Section 1
- Obtain IV access – large bore in both antecubital fossae. Send bloods for FBC, U&E, LFTs, clotting, amylase; group and save. Make the patient NBM and prescribe any necessary maintenance fluids

- Give generous analgesia – usually start with 5–10 mg morphine subcut. p.r.n., combined with an antiemetic, e.g. metoclopramide 10 mg IV
- Insert a nasogastric (NG) tube
- A catheter is useful to aid with fluid balance
- Erect CXR – often shows free air (and allows you to check the positioning of the NG tube)
- Contact a surgeon – most intervention is surgical; the surgeon can also advise on antibiotics to prescribe, and the choice of proton pump inhibitor to give the patient

Intestinal obstruction

Where the small or large bowel becomes occluded. The patient is at risk of perforation. Common causes include constipation, hernias and malignant growths.

What will the patient look like?

The patient will usually complain of a tetrad of: (i) absolute constipation; (ii) abdominal pain (colicky); (iii) bloating/distension; (iv) vomiting, which may be faeculent. The patient may also show signs of shock, and will have tinkling bowel sounds. A PR must be undertaken.

What is the immediate management?
- ABCDE – see Section 1
- Obtain IV access, with bloods sent for FBC, U&E, LFTs, clotting, amylase; group and save
- Obtain a quick history: when were the bowels last opened, when did the patient last eat, any previous abdominal surgery? Examine the patient fully, remembering to check for evidence of herniae
- Start IV fluids – e.g. 1 L normal saline 4-hourly; be guided by the clinical condition, urine output and basic observations
- Consider starting an anti-emetic, e.g cyclizine
- Make NBM and insert NG tube to aid with decompression when the obstruction is proximal to a competent ileocaecal valve
- Request an urgent AXR and erect CXR. Dilated small bowel is distinguished from dilated large bowel on AXR by the lines visible spanning the bowel. In small bowel obstruction 'valvulae conniventes' go all the way across the bowel, whereas in large bowel obstruction 'haustrae' go only part of the way across
- Call senior staff as the patient may require further imaging and surgery

Renal colic

A stone in the renal tract often causing significant, yet episodic, pain.

What will the patient look like?

Unwell with significant unilateral pain, which classically radiates 'from loin to groin'. The patient may also be nauseous and may vomit. Passing urine may hurt, and there may be haematuria.

What is the immediate management?
- Obtain IV access; take blood for FBC, U&E, amylase, calcium
- Give analgesia – both regular paracetamol and NSAIDs

- Obtain a urine sample – check for blood and β-hCG (i.e. pregnancy test)
- If febrile, consider giving antibiotics (discuss with pharmacist for local guidelines)
- Call senior staff, who will be able to advise on local imaging policy, which may be a plain X-ray, CT or USS

Ectopic pregnancy

A fetus that develops outside the womb, often in the Fallopian tube, usually 5–8 weeks after the last period.

What will the patient look like?
Female of childbearing age with abdominal pain – usually in one of the iliac fossae, and may report vaginal bleeding. The patient may be in shock. Do not exclude in patients with previous tubal ligation/coil *in situ*.

What is the immediate management?
- Obtain IV access – send bloods for FBC, U&E, β-hCG; group and save, LFTs (as methotrexate may be a treatment option).
- Give fluids (normal saline) if patient is shocked to maintain BP
- Conduct a urinary pregnancy test, and send off a urine sample to the lab for confirmation
- A trans-vaginal USS can confirm the diagnosis
- Contact the on-call gynaecologist urgently

Acute cholecystitis

Inflammation of the gallbladder wall, often caused by the presence of a stone (or other obstruction) which interrupts the flow of bile from the gallbladder.

What will the patient look like?
The patient will complain of pain in the RUQ or epigastrium, which may be referred to the tip of the right shoulder. The patient is often nauseous and may vomit, will be febrile, and will usually be positive for Murphy's sign (two fingers are pressed over the RUQ and inspiration is interrupted by pain).

What is the immediate management?
- Obtain IV access; send blood for FBC, U&E, LFTs, amylase; group and save
- NBM; give maintenance fluids
- Give analgesia – regular paracetamol/co-codamol plus p.r.n. morphine
- Request an abdominal USS
- Liaise with the surgeons; some will want to operate early, others will prefer a delayed procedure several weeks later. Ask which antibiotics you should commence

Constipation

One of the commonest causes of abdominal pain among in-patients, often due to poor hospital food, not getting enough fluids, and opiate-based medications.

What will the patient look like?

The patient will not have opened the bowels for several days and will now be either constipated or complaining of diarrhoea (overflow). The abdomen will feel full and will be uncomfortable when palpated. A PR may reveal faecal impaction.

What is the immediate management?

- Check the patient is stable
- Take a brief history: when were the bowels last opened; any vomiting/ nausea (?obstruction); what medications; what food and drinks; does the patient normally take laxatives; any recent weight loss (?malignancy); any prior bowel problems; any changes in bowel habit?
- Examine the patient's fluid status, and give IV fluids or encourage oral intake where necessary
- Check the latest blood tests – review U&Es to exclude dehydration, and review Ca^{2+} levels to ensure no hypercalcaemia
- A PR **must** be undertaken to exclude faecal impaction
- Consider non-opiate analgesic solutions
- Consider an AXR if you are concerned about obstruction
- Prescribe a regular laxative. Senna 2 tablets o.d. plus sodium docusate 100 mg b.d. is a good starting point. The next step would be to consider an enema
- If constipation persists/is severe, discuss with senior staff; other helpful people to talk to are palliative care nurses, who are used to dealing with constipation amongst patient populations

10 The agitated patient
The aggressive patient

The patient may present as acutely aggressive if he/she is confused, anxious, delirious or tired. There may be an organic cause for the aggression.

What will the patient look like?
The patient will usually be angry or upset, and behaviour may appear odd.

What is the immediate management?
- Firstly, think of your own safety and that of others. Get appropriate help *before* getting into an unfortunate situation. Good people to ask for help are security staff and medical colleagues. If you are still worried for your personal safety, do not put yourself at risk
- When approaching an aggressive patient, make sure that you keep yourself between the patient and the door
- Before approaching the patient, review the latest obs and bloods – the patient may well be delirious and therefore require medical management of the underlying infection – an MSU would be useful... if obtainable!
- Introduce yourself, giving your name, and ask the patient to sit down to discuss matters
- Explore the patient's reasons for their current mental state – are they known to be under psychiatric services? Are they angry with having to wait to be seen? Are they intoxicated?
- Try to answer any concerns, apologising where necessary. Do not enter into debate with the patient, who is probably not in a rational frame of mind
- If matters deteriorate, consider contacting security staff
- If the patient becomes a risk to themself or others, emergency sedation may be necessary; prescribing these drugs to appease nursing staff is not ethical and should not be done:
  lorazepam 0.5–1 mg subcut. or orally **or**
  haloperidol (contraindicated in Parkinson's) 2 mg subcut. or orally
  If no effect after ~10 mins, consider repeating the dose
- Ensure the patient is in an area where they can be monitored, especially due to the risk of hypoxia from a reduced respiratory drive that the above drugs can cause

The confused patient

A range of conditions can cause confusion, but the commonest cause by far is infection. It is important to exclude rare, yet serious, causes, such as cerebral infarction, hypoxia, and meningitis.

What will the patient look like?
The patient may well appear septic, demonstrated by tachycardia, hypotension, tachypnoea and a high temperature. They will be disorientated, and confused.

What is the immediate management?

- Ensure the patient is stable
- Before approaching the patient, review the latest obs and bloods for evidence of infection; remember that some elderly patients may not have an obvious pyrexia with infection
- Reassurance is required – moving the patient nearer to the nursing station in a room that is well-lit is a good start. Try to allow the patient access to a clock, and if there are any photographs of the patient's relatives, it is a good idea to put these up
- Take a brief history; a supplementary historian would be useful – ask the nursing staff or any relatives. It is often useful to contact the people who the patient lives with, e.g. a spouse or nursing home staff
- Ask about any previous problems with memory
- Conduct an AMTS – a score of <8 signifies cognitive impairment
- Consider an ABG to exclude hypoxia/hypercapnia as a cause
- Undertake a septic screen:
  - dip the urine, and send off for culture
  - request a CXR
  - check cannulation sites
  - take blood for FBC (esp. WCC), U&E, LFTs, CRP, and cultures. Also consider TFTs and calcium
  - send off a stool sample for culture
- If the patient becomes aggressive or very upset, sedation *may* be required, but first undertake the non-pharmacological methods above
- If sedation is required, begin with 0.5 mg lorazepam p.o.; do not use medications as a substitute for good nursing care
- The most important thing is to treat the underlying cause – ask for help if you get stuck

11 Emergency drug doses

Drug	Dose	Route	Covered in Section:
Activated charcoal	50 g diluted in water	PO	Metabolic emergencies
Actrapid®	10 units in 50 mL 50% dextrose over 10 mins	IV	Hyperkalaemia
Adrenaline	0.5 mg (0.5 mL 1 : 1000) 1 mg (10 mL 1 : 10,000 or 1 mL 1 : 1.000)	IM IV	Anaphylaxis Cardiac arrest
Aspirin	300 mg	PO	Stroke (ischaemic) ACS
Calcium gluconate	10 mL 10% + flush over 2 mins	IV	Hyperkalaemia
Cefuroxime	1.5 g tds	IV	Acute appendicitis
Chlorpheniramine	10 mg	IV	Anaphylaxis
Clopidogrel	300 mg loading dose, then 75 mg daily	PO	ACS
Cyclizine	50 mg	PO/IV/IM	Acute pancreatitis
Dextrose	200 mL 20% (preferably), or 50 mL 50% + flush	IV	Hypoglycaemia
Diazepam	5–10 mg	PR	Status epilepticus
Dipyridamole MR	200 mg	PO	Stroke (ischaemic)
Enoxaparin	1.5 mg/kg 1 mg/kg b.d.	SUBCUT SUBCUT	Pulmonary embolism ACS
Furosemide	40–80 mg	IV	Acute left ventricular failure
GTN spray	2 puffs	SUBLINGUAL	Acute left ventricular failure ACS
Haloperidol	2 mg	SUBCUT / PO	The agitated patient
Hydrocortisone	100 mg 200 mg	IV IV	Acute asthma Anaphylaxis
Ipratropium	0.5 mg	NEB	Acute asthma Pneumonia
Lorazepam	2–4 mg 0.5–1 mg	IV SUBCUT/PO	Status epilepticus The agitated patient
Magnesium sulphate	1.2–2 g over 20 mins	IV	Acute asthma
Metoclopramide	10 mg	IV	Pulmonary embolism ACS Acute aortic dissection Perforated peptic ulcer
Metronidazole	500 mg tds	IV	Acute appendicitis
Morphine	10 mg	IV	Pulmonary embolism ACS Acute aortic dissection Perforated peptic ulcer
Naloxone	400 µg; may need to be repeated if GCS falls	IV/IM	Opiate overdose
Parvolex®	Prescribe by weight		Paracetamol overdose
Piriton®	10 mg	IV	Anaphylaxis
Prednisolone	40 mg 30 mg	PO PO	Acute asthma Pneumonia
Salbutamol	5 mg	NEB	Acute asthma Pneumonia
Senna	2 tablets	PO	Constipation
Simvastatin	40 mg	PO	ACS
Sodium docusate	100 mg	PO	Constipation

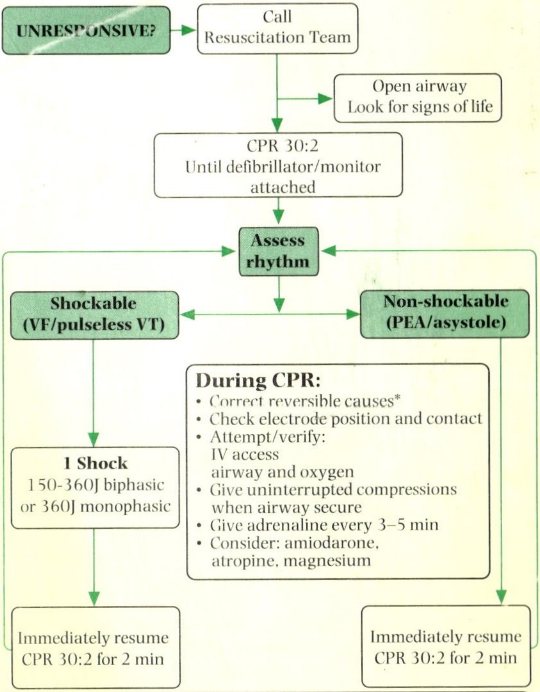

```
┌─────────────────┐      ┌─────────────────┐
│ UNRESPONSIVE?   │─────▶│ Call            │
└─────────────────┘      │ Resuscitation   │
                         │ Team            │
                         └─────────────────┘
```

UNRESPONSIVE? → Call Resuscitation Team

Open airway
Look for signs of life

CPR 30:2
Until defibrillator/monitor
attached

Assess rhythm

Shockable (VF/pulseless VT)

Non-shockable (PEA/asystole)

During CPR:
- Correct reversible causes*
- Check electrode position and contact
- Attempt/verify:
  IV access
  airway and oxygen
- Give uninterrupted compressions
  when airway secure
- Give adrenaline every 3–5 min
- Consider: amiodarone,
  atropine, magnesium

1 Shock
150-360J biphasic
or 360J monophasic

Immediately resume
CPR 30:2 for 2 min

Immediately resume
CPR 30:2 for 2 min

*Reversible causes
Hypoxia, hypovolaemia, hypo/hyperkalaemia/metabolic,
hypothermia, tension pneumothorax, tamponade, cardiac,
toxins, thrombosis (coronary or pulmonary)

Courtesy of the Resuscitation Council (UK)

ISBN 978-140519357-3

9 781405 193573

WILEY-BLACKWELL

A John Wiley & Sons, Ltd., Publication